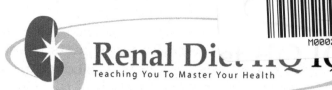

Renal Diet HQ IQ
Teaching You To Master Your Health

Eating Out On a Kidney Diet:

Pre-dialysis and Diabetes

Ways To Enjoy Your Favorite Foods

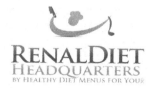

RENALDIET
HEADQUARTERS
BY HEALTHY DIET MENUS FOR YOU!

PURPOSE AND INTRODUCTION

What I have found through the emails and requests of my readers is that it is difficult to find information about a pre-dialysis kidney diet that is actionable. I want you to know that is what I intend to provide in all my books. They all fit a stage 2 – 5 kidney disease patient.

I wrote this book with you in mind: the person with kidney problems who does not know where to start or can't seem to get the answers that you need from other sources. This book will provide information that is applicable to a predialysis kidney disease diet.

Who am I? I am a registered dietitian in the USA who has been working with kidney patients for my entire 15 + years of experience. Find all my books on Amazon on my author page: http://www.amazon.com/Mathea-Ford/e/B008E1E7IS/

My goals are simple – to give some answers and to create an understanding of what is typical. It will not necessarily be what happens in your case, as everyone is an individual. I may simplify things in an effort to write them so that I feel you can learn the most from the information. This may mean that I don't say the exact things that your doctor would say. If you don't understand, please ask your doctor.

I want you to know, I am not a medical doctor and I am not aware of your particular condition. Information in this book is current as of publication, but may or may not have changed. This book is not meant to substitute for medical treatment for you, your friends, your caregivers, or your family members. You should not base treatment decisions solely on what is contained in this book. Develop your treatment plan with your doctors, nurses and the other medical professionals on your team. I recommend that you double-check any information with your medical team to verify if it applies to you.

In other words, I am not responsible for your medical care. I am providing this book for information and entertainment purposes, not medical diagnoses. Please consult with your doctor about any questions that you have about your particular case.

TABLE OF CONTENTS

GOALS OF KIDNEY DISEASE MANAGEMENT WHEN EATING OUT

Depending on the stage of your kidney failure, restrictions are more concrete than other times. If you are in stage 2 kidney failure, with a eGFR between 60-89, you should find ways to lower sodium intake but increase your intake of all kinds of vegetables and not worry so much about potassium and phosphorus. As you enter stage 4, with an eGFR of 15-29, you will need to know what foods are high in potassium and avoid them in your meals, as well as closely watch the salt in the food you eat. So this book is for a range of people, but you need to use the information based on your stage of kidney failure.

It is unfortunate that many kidney patients just stop eating out because we all enjoy the chance to socialize and "go out". While it's not something kidney patients can do all the time, but it can be done. The hesitation comes with the unknown element of having someone else prepare the food and the fear we have of getting worse or making a huge mistake! You might have to accept some unknown in eating out, but you should find a way to get out into the wild!

When you eat out, you are finding a balance between convenience and diet. You are eating out for pleasure, because you are with friends, or because you are just tired of eating at home. The end result is the same and you must make some choices.

In most cases, you won't have all of the information you would know at home. Many restaurants and fast food places provide the "required" information that you would find on a label. Potassium and phosphorus are not on the label. You are working with limited information which is why you should follow the directions in this guide.

Don't be tempted by the pretty pictures on the menu or the specials that the server tells you about. Many times, they are not good choices because they contain additional ingredients that make them higher in sodium. Stick to the plan that you had when you left home. Follow the "My Plate" guidelines – ¼ meat, ¼ starch, and ½ of your plate as vegetables (low potassium). Then you will be full and healthy. Portion control is very important, so make sure you know what a portion amount is of the food you want!

LIMIT YOUR PORTION SIZE

Many times, restaurant serving sizes are too large for even a person with normally functioning kidneys. You look at the regular meals and most of them contain entrees with at least 8-20 ounces of meat. What we think of as "normal" portion sizes now are almost 2 times as big as they were just 10-15 years ago. Supersizing our meals has lead to more health problems and issues than we even know. So, be aware that you are starting with a larger meal than normal.

If you eat out once in a while (monthly) you might be ok to eat a little more. But many people eat out 1-2 times per week. You have to be as diligent with those meals as you are in your normal everyday meals that you make at home. You can't ignore the portion size like you have no control. <u>You have complete control over how much you eat and what you order. So, you are in charge!</u>

What happens at restaurants is called "portion distortion". If you have been on enough diets or watching what you eat for very long, you know how easy it is to be tempted to "eyeball" the portion size. If you were to use a scale or measuring device, how often would your "guess" be right? Not very often. It's very difficult to measure with your eyes.

Let me give you some examples so you can make sure that you don't fall into this trap.

1. When you order a pizza, you usually order a large, right? You should have only 2 slices as a serving – especially since this one is high in salt. But the good thing about a pizza is that it is completely customizable.

2. But what about those chips they serve before the meal at a Mexican restaurant? A serving is 12 of them. Not the 30 or so that you eat before the meal comes. If you want the chips, count out 12 of them and that is all you eat. Send the bowl away from the table.

3. A bagel seems like a good choice... but it's usually at least 3 servings if you eat all of it. And you add the cream cheese – wow, you are getting into some major over-portioning.

4. Drinking a clear soda? If you pick up a 20 ounce drink from the machine, you are looking at about 300 calories. A serving is more like 8 ounces which is around 100 calories.

5. A serving of French fries is about 10-13 fries – even less than the small serving of fries – more like the McDonald's ® new French fries in their kids meal.

Ok, now you know. You need to make sure that your portions stay in line with what you should be eating all the time. We will talk later about specific foods and restaurants, but make sure you always stick to a smaller portion size. Look for words that indicate the meal is being "enlarged" such as – combo, deluxe, supreme, supersize, all you can eat, Value meal... All of those indicate you are going to get more like an entrée, side and beverage. Make sure you can choose the side dish, and pay attention to the portion sizes.

Finally, eat slowly. It really is true that it takes about 20 minutes for your stomach to signal your brain that you are full, so the slower you eat, the more time you have to socialize and know if you are really full. That keeps you from feeling overly full and stuffed as well.

Action step: Instead of just assuming you can't get another size – ASK! Ask your server if they have a lunch size portion, or take ½ home with you, or other ways to decrease the portion. Sometimes, just because something has the word "Value" on it, does not mean it is a value for your heart or your kidneys. You may pay a little more for a different meal so you can eat less.

Some examples of asking for special sizes might be to request something "on the side" or with no added salt. You might ask about how the food is prepared – many times the entrée is grilled and during grilling the staff brushes it with butter or other sauce. As them to tell you if they do that. If you can share with another person at the table, please do. Many times all you have to do is ask at the table, "would anyone mind sharing a meal with me?"

Also, know your serving amounts or "allowances". If you are supposed to eat 3 ounces meat, one fruit, 2 vegetables, 1 starch, etc – then do your best to build a meal that fits that pattern.

FOCUS ON THE AMOUNT OF PROTEIN BEING SERVED

The second most important thing that you have to do as part of eating out is watch the portion size of the protein. Now, you should watch the overall amounts of your meal as far as calories, but protein is your main concern since it has so much ability to affect your health in negative ways very quickly.

So make sure you know that a 3 ounce serving of meat is the size of a deck of cards. Know that, and don't let your "eyes" weigh it instead. Err on the side of making it a smaller portion. Ask for the child size portion or ask a server what size portion the main entrée item is so you can determine if you need to cut it down. Protein is also contained in cheese and cream sauce, as well as nuts and eggs. Plus, many vegetarian meals that contain beans and lentils have protein in them as well. The beans provide additional protein, so you need to understand how much you are getting in your serving size.

An easy way to decrease the portion size you receive it to get an appetizer instead of a full meal. You could also order ala carte. Use the children's menu. Anything to get yourself a smaller portion without tempting yourself. See the money you spend not as buying something you have to eat – you don't want to throw it away – but as spending time with others. Those meals with friends renew your soul. But don't look at the food as fulfilling a need, but just to fill your stomach for a while. Try to focus less on the food (even though you are still counting it) and more on the camaraderie. It's a wonderful thing to spend time together. That said, don't mindlessly eat without thinking about what you are eating.

Action step: Find out the amount of meat in the serving or choose a casserole dish without meat (vegetarian options are best just watch the amount of beans). Pay attention to other items that may contribute protein – cheeses, milks, and beans for example.

Another thing you can do is to substitute the meat in the meal with vegetables or starches. For example, if you found that all the entrees seem too large – you could see about eating a salad or ½ sandwich meal, or just an all vegetable plate.

KEEP THE AMOUNT OF SODIUM AT BAY

Sodium and salt are also your adversary in eating out. While potassium and phosphorus are important – and should be counted – you know that sodium is much higher in foods that are pre-prepared. Just because of the need to preserve the food and for flavor. We are accustomed to eating large amounts of salt. But, not you – on your kidney diet you have learned to survive without. And it's wonderful. You will be able to tell soon after if you have eaten too much salt.

But, you don't always know how much salt is in your meal. You CAN know – if you plan ahead and know where you are going to eat. You can check out their meals on line ahead of time, or if they are a national chain restaurant they might have brochures with that information right there in the business. But, if you don't know – you can do a few things to lower the sodium right now before you eat.

1. <u>Ask how the food is prepared</u>. If you are with a large group and you want to know this – you might tell the wait staff that you have a special diet and need a few questions answered. Many times, they might call the manager over to answer for you so that you get the

right answer. Ask about sauces and how things are mixed together. Do they add a sauce or just marinade? What's in the marinade? Do they brush on butter when cooking, and what is cooked at the same time as this food? (why – you need to know for allergies and possibly if it could add potassium or phosphorus)

2. <u>Find out if it's possible to substitute</u>. They may buy the ingredients and create it from scratch in the restaurant and you will be fine because they can adjust what they put in the meal. But if they purchase pre-made mixes or entrees – you might have a problem. That's when you should fall back to a plain chicken breast or fish fillet that will be able to keep you "safe" even if it's not your first choice.

3. <u>Find out if they can remove certain items or leave them "on the side"</u>. Such as sauces or dressings. Then you can add a smaller amount and not affect your condition as much. Many of the sauces contain MSG or other 'sodium' type compounds, which need to be limited.

4. <u>Don't add salt at the table</u>. Your meal already has twice the salt of what you would have in a home made meal.

<u>Action Steps</u>: Prior to eating at a restaurant, go to their website and find out if they list nutritionals. Use that information to plan your meal before you go to the restaurant. Remember, planning is very helpful to you to stay on track.

Additionally, ask a lot of questions – prepare your wait staff by stating – "I have some special diet needs and I will need to know a lot about how you prepare the food I am interested in." They are more than willing to help, especially if you give them a bit of notice. And your friends should understand it may take a few more minutes for you to order.

MAKE A MEAL PLAN – DON'T JUST WAIT UNTIL THE LAST MINUTE

Ok, I have already talked a little about preparing for the meal. But, it is vital to know ahead of time what you are going to eat. You have a very special condition and you need to take good care of yourself.

Making a plan helps whether you eat out a lot or a little. Most people enjoy the company and it's just plain fun to sit around with friends and talk. But you can plan ahead by checking out the website and seeing what the menu has to offer before you even go. And remember that the reason you went in the first place is to enjoy the company of others, not necessarily to eat a lot of food. If you get any say in the choice of restaurant, choose one that will be easy to adjust meals to meet your needs – whether it's not adding certain things to the meal or ordering ala carte. If you go to a place often, they get to know you and enjoy helping you. You might want to go at a time when the staff are not necessarily busy, like early for the evening meal.

Let's talk about the plan if you eat out a lot – like you travel or you eat lunch daily at a restaurant or cafeteria as part of your job. Choose a few places to go and learn a lot about the meals they prepare. Get to know the staff and what meals you can eat. Eat more portions of vegetables and bread than meat. Read the nutritionals. I know that sounds boring – but believe me – it's one of the best ways you can plan your meals.

Lots of time, we prepare a few meals that we really like that are "comfortable" to us. We enjoy those meals and we know they are good for us. Do the same when eating out. If you are unsure what is in the food or what you can eat – choose the meal closest to a plain meat product (chicken, fish or beef) and a side of vegetables. You should be ok with that. (Also known as your "fall back" meal) Make sure the vegetables are a low potassium vegetable. You can have plain white rice or noodles with your meal too.

Just as a reminder – review your menu plan prior to going out, eat a little less that day than you normally do to leave room for your "out to eat" meal, and carefully plan what you will eat when you go out to eat.

RESOURCES YOU SHOULD USE

1. Call ahead and ask about certain foods. Call at a time when they are not busy – between meals or early in the evening meal. Ask to speak with a manager and explain what you are trying to do.
2. Review your low potassium and phosphorus foods list. You will need to keep those in mind when asking about what types of items are in a recipe and what changes can be made.
3. Choose your meal prior to going if you can. Find out what you can order and know what the nutritional information says on line about it and go in with that to eat. This helps a lot because you don't even look at the menu – no temptation.

FAST FOODS OR CONVENIENCE FOODS HAVE MORE THAN JUST A MONETARY COST

Fast food and/or convenience foods are inexpensive. Usually. Although, cooking at home is actually just as inexpensive. And better for you. But I know how much fun it can be – or just a relief – to eat out.

These foods are usually high in sodium, since they are made from pre-prepared products. They are made to be produced inexpensively and without a lot of changes.

Better choices are the child size meals at fast food or convenience places. Those are most likely the "safe" bet – except for the fries. With a child meal, you can change out the sides most of the time – with apples or a salad. Even if it's a little more, it's worth it. Also, check to see if – even at a fast food place – you can substitute the French fries for a salad. Many quick service restaurants have those choices available.

The sodium raises your blood pressure (you already know this). In general, when you eat out – regardless of the place – you are getting a lower fiber and higher fat meal. Neither of which you would like to do on a regular basis. You probably will have higher blood sugars if you have diabetes as well.

One option you have is to ask about what the food contains – MSG, added sugar, added salts. If it's a national chain restaurant you will probably be able to find this on the main website for the company.

This is the result you will get when you search for healthy restaurants. This will give you a great way to find the lower sodium choices on the menu when you need them. It shows an estimate on the prices and the healthy dining choices. While not specific for "renal diets", you can find the low sodium choices and help yourself navigate the realm of both fast foods and restaurant dining establishments.

Another option is to look on a website called
healthydiningfinder.com

Now displaying restaurants [Within 10 miles ▾] of [73165] ordered by [Price: high to low ▾] [apply]

restaurant		options	price	distance
Denny's	Denny's	13 Healthy Dining 4 Sodium Savvy 3 Kids LiveWell	$$	5.6 miles
	Chili's	8 Healthy Dining 8 Kids LiveWell	$$	6.2 miles
RED LOBSTER	Red Lobster	40 Healthy Dining 11 Sodium Savvy	$$	9.9 miles
Jack in the box	Jack in the Box	10 Healthy Dining 6 Sodium Savvy	$	6.2 miles

This picture is from their website showing an example of what
is available there. You need to go to the website and enter
your information to see what healthy dining options are
available around you.

GENERAL GUIDELINES FOR EATING OUT (WHAT TO CHOOSE)

Many places have "low sodium" or "heart healthy" meals. And using the healthy dining finder website will narrow your focus before you get to the restaurant. Ask for more information from the waiter or waitress about what is in the specific food. Most servers can tell you or refer you to someone who can.

Be careful of food that is lower in sodium – it might be higher in fat and sugars. And foods that are listed as low fat might have more salt to make up for the taste. Review the ingredients and make sure you avoid the foods that are extra-high in potassium like: beans, avocados, oranges, bananas, figs, raisins and chocolate.

Good choices are:

Low potassium vegetables and fruits

Breads (white not whole grain)

Salads

Oil and Vinegar or Lemon Juice

Grilled or Baked foods without toppings

Poor Choices are: (High in sodium)

Soups

Heavily marinated items

Cream sauces and gravies

Soy sauce or Ketchup

Salad Dressings

Deep Fried Foods

Cold Cuts, Sausage, Bacon

OTHER NOTES FOR YOU WHEN EATING OUT
Foods that are too salty may increase your thirst or cause you to retain water. Both can take a few days to recover from.

If you take any medications with meals – either insulin or phosphate binders – be sure you have those with you. You will need them.

If you "splurge" and eat too much – forgive yourself and move on. Do better next time. Sometimes you have those days – but if you let them be the majority of the time you will not be successful with managing your meal planning for kidney disease.

HAVE A STRATEGY FOR THE WEEK TO MAKE THE MOST OF YOUR MEALS

When you have special needs like those of the renal diet, it can be a daily frustration to figure out what to eat. This is why meal planning is so important for you. It also helps you plan ahead and know what you are doing. When we "plan" on the fly, it usually is not as successful as we would like. To bring about the change that you need, you should get into the "habit" of planning ahead: knowing when you are going to eat and where.

Starting with your weekly meals, make sure you know what you are going to do for the week. Choose the meals you will eat at home and the ones that you will eat "out" or at other places.

HOW TO PLAN YOUR WEEK OF MEALS

Weekly planning is best, since you can go to the grocery store one time per week and save gas and time. It's easy to take a calendar and plot out your lunches and dinners. If you like to eat the same meal for breakfast – plan it and know what you are going to eat. I would start with your work week (if you work) and write down your major events and activities.

1. Print out a calendar for the month (or just for a week). Note what dates you will be doing something – dinner with friends, holidays, travel plans. One good place to go (if you don't have a calendar) is google calendar. www.google.com/calendar You can access it anywhere and add it to your smartphone. You can put your meals on the calendar very easily.

2. Look at your breakfast first. Is there a breakfast that you really like or even just eat regularly. Breakfast is one meal most people eat the same things most of the time. Sometimes you can make this up ahead of time and have it ready to go. Like pouring your cereal the night before. If it goes with your meal pattern for the day – write it out. Track down what you need to make it for the week – eggs, juice, milk, etc.

3. Look at your evening meal. Bring up your meals for the week on the meal plan. Are there meals you really like that you want to eat more than once? Can you save part of the meal and take it for lunch the following day? What other "quick and easy" meals can you make for supper? Do you have meals that you liked from weeks before that you can make again? Based on your plans, do any nights of the week require you to eat out or away from home? How can you plan for that? Plan your meal for that day with a "sack lunch" you can take with you or plan ahead which restaurant you will go to and know what you can eat there. Either way, knowing ahead of time that you will be "out" for that meal means you can plan ahead.

4. I would recommend using an app to track your shopping list – I personally use a product called "Anylist" which is an iPhone app. I like it because it's free and I can share it with my family members. When they add to the grocery list on their phone it updates in real time on mine! Then the list is more complete when you go to the store. You can search in the android market place for a shopping list. Or you can use Remember the Milk – www.rememberthemilk.com which is available on a computer and an app in the iphone store so you can take the tasks with you. You

always can make a shopping list as well. Using a grocery list will save you money – but only if you follow it!

5. Once you know what you want to do for breakfast and dinner meals – then I recommend looking at your lunch. You will be able to use leftovers or make sandwiches from the evening meals – or at least coordinate with what you want to use. Your evening meals really help set up what you want to do for the lunch meals.

Now that you have planned the meals and know where you are going to eat them, you have a choice about what to eat. Plan where you are going to eat and choose wisely.

Other choices you might have are to keep a list of meals that you like that are quick to fix and convenient. Then you can grab that and go. Or choose some nutrition bars you can eat to snack on. Make a quick omelet or ½ sandwich and some crackers. You can put meal sized portions in the refrigerator or freezer for use later – if you live alone, you might find this the best choice to do with your meal pattern and plans for the week if you like something but the recipe is for 4-6 people. Make it and store the other 4-6 portions in the refrigerator or freezer.

Another tip is to get ready for the week with a few bags of cut up celery and carrots to carry with you on a long trip or ride so you won't get hungry and overeat. It will keep the hungry monster at bay!

General Guidelines For Meals

Good Choices for Breakfast

When eating out for breakfast, it can be very easy to stay on your diet. Most of the time, we order "a la carte" for that meal, so it's not so unusual to have a mixture of food items. Remember, you are in charge.

It's best to choose eggs that are cooked the way you like or omelets with low potassium vegetables. That way you get complete protein in your meal. You also know how much protein you receive in your meal if you know how many eggs were used (1 egg = 7 gm protein). Avoiding the salty meats like sausage and bacon to keep your intake of salt low. Occasionally, you can have a slice or two of Canadian bacon if you need some meat.

If you choose omelets, try to use low potassium vegetables and fruits even, and limit the amount of cheese or high sodium meats. You can eat the plain breads and bagels but stay away from the bran muffins or biscuits that might be high in sodium. Even French toast, waffles, and pancakes are ok and if you are not diabetic, you can eat them with regular syrup. If you are diabetic, try to find a type of sugar free syrup you like and limit the amount of starches.

Hot or cold cereals are, for the most part, perfectly fine choices for breakfast. Don't choose the bran or granola cereals if you are in late stage 3 or higher kidney failure due to the fact that they can have more potassium. Be cautious with the milk as well due to the potassium and phosphorus content, use the least amount possible. But you can add butter and a little non dairy creamer to your hot cereal to make it more flavorful.

Finally, using low potassium fruits such as apples, applesauce, grapes, pineapples and their juices are a good way to round out the meal. While you should avoid pastries every day – you can have a plain donut or sweet roll occasionally. Just skip the pastry with chocolate or nuts.

GOOD CHOICES FOR APPETIZERS & SALADS

Many times, salads are good choices for people with kidney failure because you can "create your own". You can ask the server to change the ingredients or substitute items to make a healthier salad that meets your needs. You should ask for the dressing to be on the side because it's easier to control the amount that is put on your salad. And if you don't like any of the dressings, ask for oil and vinegar to put on your salad. Put a little cracked pepper and you are good to go!

A chef salad, for example, without the ham or cheese and with the dressing on the side would make a perfect meal. Or a green salad with a 3 ounce portion of meat (fish, chicken or beef) would be an excellent meal for a person with renal failure.

Salads to avoid are those that have spinach, tomato, avocado, nuts, or beans in them. If you can have the server remove those ingredients and make your salad without them, you can eat the salad. Good ingredients in the salad are lettuce, cabbage, beets, cauliflower, celery, cucumber, onions, green peas, sprouts, and peppers. Those salads you can create on a salad bar would be optimal so you can add extra of the ingredients you know are healthier for your diet.

Another salad to avoid is potato salad due to the potassium levels, and any sort of salad with olives and pickles due to the sodium. Fruit salads and gelatin salads that have some canned fruit in them can be healthy foods for your meal. Canned peaches, pears and pineapple are some of the best sides to have if you want a salad for your main course.

Appetizers can be an excellent way to have a small meal instead of choosing a larger entrée and dividing it in half. But watch out for the higher concentration of fried and salty foods in this category. Eat the foods that are baked and have a smaller amount of meat – like tostadas or small salads. Avoid the items with cheese like fried mozzarella sticks and cottage cheese. Soups and smoked meats are very high in sodium, so leave them off your meal as well.

GOOD CHOICES FOR LUNCH AND SUPPER ENTREES

Now, for the main course. You have looked forward to your night out with friends or a significant other, and you want something to eat. Where should you start to look?

In a restaurant, by their very nature, the portions are larger than you would normally make at home. At this point, you probably know how much you are used to eating, so don't overdo it. Putting part of the meal to the side at the beginning is a great way to avoid any issues. But you also need to start with a great meal. Stick to about 3 ounces of meat at this meal. A grilled meat is the best choice and make sure to tell the serving staff that you don't want them to add any sauces when cooking it. Have them put the gravies and sauces on the side, and ask for lemon or lime to squeeze on your meat to bring out the natural flavors.

As much as you might like them, avoid any sort of casseroles as they are often made with high sodium soups that can add too much salt to your daily allowance. Other sauces that add salt are soy and Worcestershire sauce. Read the label on any sauces brought to the table, and use the natural lemon or lime to bring out the flavor.

Many times plain beef or chicken is best to be safe. You can also choose kabobs with your allowed vegetables (onions and peppers are usually fine), just make sure they don't add a sauce when cooking. If you happen to be in a deli, a sandwich on white is fine with no cheese and using roast beef, turkey, or chicken. Avoid the bacon, canned tuna, and Reuben style sandwiches.

BEST CHOICES FOR SIDE DISHES AT MEALS

The more you eat the foods on your diet, the more you will be able to tell what items you are able to eat without much thought. For the most part, you are still continuing to choose low potassium vegetables like asparagus, cabbage, carrots, corn, green peas, zucchini, coleslaw and salads. Avoid potatoes and sweet potatoes, as well as other high potassium vegetables like tomatoes, spinach, collard greens, acorn squash, and artichokes.

The best starches to complete your meals are noodles, rice, pasta, or white breads. Make sure you understand the portion amount if you are a diabetic, but ask if your server can replace the potatoes with rice as a first step. Most restaurants will allow you to do this.

WHAT TO ORDER FOR BEVERAGES

Beverages can have detrimental consequences to your diet as well. You need to watch the amount of potassium and phosphorus in drinks. And if you are on a fluid restriction (later stages of kidney disease and some types of dialysis), you should make a concerted effort to remove the glasses or make sure that your glass is not refilled so you can stick to your restriction. Once you are no longer making urine, you need to keep your fluid at a level that your nephrologist will instruct you about.

Drinks that you can have include apple juice, lemonade, water and non-cola drinks (clear) such as 7-up®, Sprite®, or Ginger Ale. You can also have a limited amount of coffee unless it's decaffeinated. Try to limit your intake of caffeine because of the heart problems you are already prone to as a renal patient. You should avoid milk based drinks – including milk shakes – due to phosphorus amounts. And if you want to have an alcoholic drink, stick to red or white wine to reduce potassium intake. Don't drink mixed drinks with tomato juice or milk based mixers.

WHAT TO ORDER FOR DESSERTS

Now onto the best part of the meal. Dessert! When you are done eating the main course (whether it is a salad, appetizer, or main entrée), you should look forward to this part of your meal.

Ask for a clear definition of what is in the dessert. Even if you think you know, ask. Each place could be a little different. Look for a simple dessert. One that doesn't have a lot of sauces and nuances. Just something like angel food cake, pound cake, or white cake with whipped cream icing. Or a couple of cookies like shortbread cookies, lemon crème cookies, or sugar cookies. Any sort of pie that is made with low potassium fruits, like apple, blueberry, cherry, or strawberry, would also be a good choice.

What you want to avoid in the desserts is: chocolate and nuts. You can have fruit ices (they are fluid if you are counting) but

> not the ice cream (more of the milk based products). Unless you share it with a friend, you should not choose the chocolate
> cream, banana cream, minced meat, pecan, pumpkin, or sweet
> potato pies. And cheesecake is also to be avoided. Again, keep it simple and know what all the ingredients are in the product you eat so you can make a healthier choice.

WHAT OTHER OPTIONS DO I HAVE FOR EATING OUTSIDE OF THE HOME?

You have many options – some you may have thought of and some you have not. You will see that I emphasize using your resources to make the food at home and take it along instead of purchasing food out to eat – the control you have over the ingredients and what is good for you is worth the extra time.

1. <u>Take your lunch with you</u>. This requires you to plan ahead and know what you want to do. It may require you to have a cooler. I have known many people who drive for hours to go places or drive for a living (taxi, etc) that take a cooler with snacks and their meal. They use things like, low potassium fruits and vegetables for snacks and crackers. They make a lunch using their pattern – preparing a healthy sandwich and side dish or something they can heat up when they get there. Even a jelly and butter sandwich (my kids favorite) can be a good choice on the road.

2. <u>Pick a couple of meals that you like to eat and repeat them</u>. I know it sounds boring, but it's the best way to make sure that you are getting it right. I have said this before but it bears repeating – you should find what works that you like and keep on doing that.

3. <u>Use leftovers from the night before</u>. Be intentional about cooking – make an extra serving to take to work the next day or have for lunch. Using leftovers is smart because you cooked one time and were able to use it twice, which is a great use of time. Especially if you are feeling some fatigue, it is very helpful to have food

prepared ahead of time. Another version of using leftovers is to cook ahead and make more portions, and then divide them into meal sized containers for use later in the week or to be frozen – this saves your time and energy.

4. <u>Take a nutrition bar with you</u>. A nutrition bar is a quick meal or snack that you can take with you instead of a full meal. It typically contains high amounts of certain nutrients. But some nutrition bars are better than others for people with kidney failure. For example, Kashi Go Lean Crunchy Chocolate Pretzel Bars are great for kidney failure, because they can be very filling at 160 calories but only have 5 grams of protein. They can help to hold you over to the next meal with extra fiber in the bar and not excessive amounts of protein. Luna bars in many flavors can be healthy for kidney failure too – they only contain about 10 gm of protein.

5. <u>Choose between eating at a restaurant and a fast food place.</u> I would choose each for different reasons. If you are in a hurry and can find the information on the fast food restaurant nutritional guides – you could choose wisely at a fast food place and still maintain your diet. If you go to a restaurant – ask lots of questions and stick to the "safe" foods list.

Specialty Advice for Restaurants

Chinese Cuisine

Ask which foods contain MSG or (monosodium glutamate), soy or fish sauce. These are high in sodium and should be avoided or request that they prepare the food with little to none of it. Don't add soy sauce at the table, either. It's very high in sodium and will keep you from eating a healthy low sodium meal.

Stay away from soups – they contain a high amount of sodium and may cause you to retain fluid

Ask how the food is prepared and ask if they can prepare your food individually instead of in bulk.

Don't add the soy sauce provided at the table, many places have a hot pepper oil that can be used to add flavor to the recipes at the table.

Eat the plain rice or brown rice instead of the fried rice – it will have lower sodium.

Choose lower potassium vegetables in your meal – ask for snow peas, string beans, water chestnuts, bean sprouts, and bok choy. Ask for your stir fry sauces on the side.

If you are limiting your fluid intake – make sure you don't drink too much tea.

French Cuisine

These may use a lot of cream and butter in recipes – ask what they use and be sure they don't add extra salt to the meal.

Avoid lots of cream or cheese sauces – they have extra sodium and are possibly higher in potassium

Avoid the potatoes – but choose the lower potassium fruits and vegetables for your side dishes

You can possibly eat the bread with some oil, as it should be low in sodium, potassium and phosphorus

Use a light version of dressing or vinegar and oil dressing for your salad

Desserts can be yummy sorbets, fruit, cakes, and meringues but don't eat the additional chocolate and heavy cream sauces that might be on them, ask for them on the side.

MEXICAN CUISINE

While the chips might be ok at the beginning of the meal, they are probably really salty. It's best to avoid them – or limit yourself to just a couple. Extra salt is not what you need!

Choose a single item – not a meal. The beans that are a side dish are high in potassium and should be avoided. Choose double rice or vegetables if you want a meal.

Good a la carte items are : tacos, tostados and fajitas. Without the salsa and limited on the sour cream.

Even the green salsa, "salsa verde", is made from tomatoes. And the guacamole is from avocado which is also high in potassium. You will need to eat the chips plain.

Often they have marinated vegetables which are a good choice – the onions, carrots and jalapenos are good vegetables as long as you don't have a fluid restriction.

Tortillas are good bread items, and not too high in sodium or potassium. If you are a diabetic, watch your portions on them. Otherwise, they make a great filler without extra sodium and potassium. Corn tortillas are better than flour tortillas but both are good for you.

Dessert can be some simple fruit or a sopapilla. This fried dough is served with honey and sugar and is made from tortillas. They do have a lot of fat, so don't overdo it, but you can have a dessert item. Maybe you can split one with a friend.

ASIAN / INDIAN CUISINE

Indian meals have many vegetarian choices. You may have to ask, but you can get a lot of good foods that have no additional meat – which lowers the amount of protein. Careful of the beans they may contain, though, and the spices.

Asian Indian cuisine is very flavorful, and you can try masala, tandoori and curry recipes that provide a lot of color and flavor with little sodium but make sure you don't overload on fluid.

Yogurt is a popular side dish, but should be limited due to its phosphorus levels, so choose a small taste instead of a bowl.

Indian breads – whether fried, baked, or roasted – are good side dishes to your meal. Use caution if you have diabetes with the portion sizes.

Ask which vegetables are included in the dish, and see if you can make substitutions for lower potassium vegetable servings.

Desserts often contain milk, be sure to choose with that in mind and ask your server about ingredients. They tend to be very understanding of special diets.

ITALIAN CUISINE

The antipasto appetizer that comes at the beginning of the meal is full of sodium and meat. It would be a good thing to skip. Limit your consumption of cheeses, olives, and cured meats because they are also high in sodium.

Any soups on the menu are likely high in sodium, so you should choose a salad with oil and vinegar dressing for your appetizer.

The Italian bread is good to eat (use caution if you are a diabetic), and you are given oil to dip the slices in which is a good choice and low in saturated fat.

Look for a butter or pesto sauce to use instead of the tomato based sauce that many of the dishes have. You should be able to substitute items. The tomato soup is high in potassium.

Many Italian restaurants offer pizza, so substitute the tomato sauce with a butter or plain sauce and choose vegetables that fit in your diet with some cheese. You may use a tablespoon of shredded Parmesan or Romano cheese to flavor – and the pepper flakes may be used liberally. The best part about a pizza is that they are made to personalize!

Italian ices are usually a good bet for dessert.

JAPANESE CUISINE

Soups are to be avoided, as they are very salty. Even a soup that looks like just a broth soup is filled with salt.

Ask which items on the menu contain MSG and avoid them. Also avoid using the soy sauce at the table.

Sushi is a good bet! It is usually made with fresh ingredients and healthy items. Be cautious with raw or uncooked items as they may cause you to have food borne illnesses. Ask the chef if the fish is cooked or raw, and choose cooked fish.

Eat the kabobs, or yakitori (food on skewers). Also tempura vegetables are a healthy choice even though they are dipped and fried – just make sure the sauce is not high in sodium.

Watch out for tofu or soy bean curd. It is used a lot in Japanese foods, and may have added soy sauce to enhance the flavor.

Japanese steak houses offer good choices of healthy foods and since you can request the food be prepared in a specific way you can eat healthier. Just watch the portion size.

FAST FOOD CHOICES

Many condiments are high in sodium – ketchup, BBQ sauce, and soy sauce. Avoid or limit the use of them.

Plan ahead and choose the "junior" or kids meal – just avoid the French fries and eat a side salad instead if you can.

You can easily look up sodium and protein amounts for recipes on the website for the restaurant.

Choose the roast beef or turkey sandwich instead of bacon and cheese at sandwich shops.

Eat grilled or broiled chicken items instead of fried and breaded items.

Eat more of the coleslaw, lettuce salads, and macaroni salad instead of the pickles and tomatoes

Drink the clear sodas, lemonade, and tea or coffee.

RECOMMENDATIONS FOR LOWER SODIUM FAST FOOD OPTIONS

Based on current data from the following companies, I am providing the nutrition information that should help with coming up with a quality decision on what to eat. This does not qualify as an endorsement of any of these brands.

As far as potassium and phosphorus, the restaurant or fast food companies do not publish those numbers. In each section, I provide a healthy similar recipe so you can make a comparable meal at home. While it is not an exact replica, it should be close and allow you to enjoy that taste without a major adjustment to your day because you ate out at a restaurant and don't know how much potassium and phosphorus you had in your meal.

You can take the numbers from this chart and generalize the information slightly. What I mean by that is, if you have another taco that has the same ingredients as the company listed's taco, you could feel somewhat confident that the information is close to that listed. The science is not exact and individual variation makes a difference as well.

I have chosen the healthiest and lowest sodium products for you to start with. These meals are the lowest sodium meals that restaurant has. Your main goals with eating out are controlling the protein and sodium content because you don't know the potassium and phosphorus levels for foods, but you can control the items you choose for potassium and phosphorus knowing what you have learned in this book.

After each section of nutritionals, I have included some adjusted recipes that are "similar" to what you might eat at that restaurant for you to try at home.

McDonalds ® as of 4-8-2013

http://nutrition.mcdonalds.com/getnutrition/nutritionfacts.pdf

Product	Calories	Sodium	Protein
Hamburger	250	480	12
Cheeseburger	300	680	15
Grilled Onion Cheddar	310	660	15
Filet O Fish	390	590	15
Chipotle BBQ Snack Wrap (Grilled)	250	670	16
Honey Mustard Snack Wrap (Grilled)	250	650	16
Mac Snack Wrap	330	670	14
Ranch Snack Wrap	270	700	16
Chicken McNugget (4 pc)	190	360	9
Chicken McNugget (6 pc)	280	540	13
Fish McBites (Happy Meal sz)	170	300	8
Fish McBites (regular size)	370	630	17
Bacon Ranch Salad Chicken (Grilled) no dressing	230	700	30
Bacon Ranch Salad – No Chicken	140	300	9
Caesar Salad with Grilled Chicken (no dressing)	190	580	27
Caesar Salad – No Chicken	90	180	7
Southwest Salad with Grilled Chicken (no dressing)	290	650	27
Southwest Salad – No Chicken	140	150	6
Side Salad	20	10	1
Fruit and Yogurt Parfait	150	70	4
Hotcakes	350	590	15
Hashbrowns	150	310	1
Fruit and Maple Oatmeal	290	160	5
Fruit and Maple Oatmeal (no Brown sugar)	260	115	5
Apple Slices	15	0	0
Creamy Southwest Dressing	100	340	1
Creamy Caesar Dressing	190	500	2
Low Fat Balsamic Vinaigrette	35	420	0
Low Fat Family Italian Dressing	50	390	1
Ranch Dressing	170	30	1
Ketchup Packet	10	100	0
BBQ Sauce Packet	50	260	0
Sweet N Sour Sauce	50	150	0

I know it's not always easy or convenient to cook from home, but I have taken a couple of the meals that you might go out for, found the recipe, and created a recipe that you can use as part of your meal planning at home. For McDonalds®, I chose a hamburger and a Southwest Chicken Salad.

McDONALD'S® STYLE HAMBURGER
Ingredients:

1.	Ground Beef, 90% lean, Raw	2 ounces
2.	Hamburger bun, White	1 Hamburger bun
3.	Catsup, Regular	1 Tablespoon
4.	Mustard, Regular	½ Teaspoon
5.	Chopped Onions, Minced	½ Tablespoon

Using lean ground beef, roll just the ground beef into a ball and press flat on wax paper until it's only about ¼ inch thick. In a medium pan, brown the insides of the bun over medium heat. After the bun is cooked, set it aside. Cook the hamburger meat for about 2 minutes per side and add pepper if desired to each side of burger.

On the top bun, add the catsup, mustard, and onion. Add the cooked hamburger then finish by putting the hamburger together with the bottom bun. Microwave for 10-15 seconds. You are ready to eat.

NUTRITIONAL ANALYSIS PER SERVING: Calories: 237, Protein 15.7 gm, Carbohydrate 25.6 gm, Fiber 1.1 gm, Fat 7.6 gm, Saturated Fat 2.56 gm, Phosphorus 139 mg, Potassium 288 mg, Sodium 439 mg.

SOUTHWEST CHICKEN SALAD

Ingredients:

1.	Chicken Breast, Boneless, Raw	3 ounces
2.	Mixed Salad Greens, Raw	1 cup
3.	Frozen Corn	¼ cup
4.	Black Beans, Canned	¼ cup
5.	Lime Juice	2 Tablespoons
6.	Carrots, Chopped	¼ cup
7.	Cheddar Cheese	½ ounce
8.	Tortilla Chips, Plain (about 8)	½ ounce
9.	Cilantro	1 sprig
10.	Olive Oil	2 Tablespoons
11.	Vinegar, Red Wine	1 Tablespoon

Bake or grill plain chicken breast until done. You may pound chicken breast flat if desired. You can add Mrs. Dash or other salt free seasoning while cooking to add flavor. Chop chicken breast into strips and set aside. Add salad mix to bowl. Warm corn in microwave if frozen, and add to salad along with black beans, cheese, carrots and lime juice. Toss together if desired. Crunch tortilla chips and add to salad.

Place chicken on top of salad mixed greens. Chop cilantro and add to oil and vinegar then mix thoroughly. Add to salad and toss. Enjoy. (While the dressing is not creamy like the restaurant, it makes this salad very flavorful.

NUTRITIONAL ANALYSIS PER SERVING: Calories 558, Protein 27 gm, Carbohydrate 29 gm, Fiber 5.6 gm, Fat 38 gm, Saturated Fat 7.9 gm, Phosphorus 375 mg, Potassium 819 mg, Sodium 415.3 mg.

(MEXICAN) TACO BELL® as of 4/15/13

http://www.tacobell.com/nutrition/information

Product	Calories	Sodium	Protein
Chalupa Supreme – Chicken	340	530	16
Chalupa Supreme – Steak	350	500	16
Bacon AM Griller	250	610	12
Hashbrowns	170	260	1
Sausage AM Griller	240	470	9
Fresco Crunchy Taco	140	290	6
Fresco Grilled Steak Soft Taco	160	430	11
Fresco Soft Taco	170	500	8
Gordita Supreme – Chicken	270	510	16
Gordita Supreme – Steak	280	480	16
Cheesy Nachos	270	280	3
Nachos Supreme	430	690	12
Pintos & Cheese	180	560	9
Chicken Soft Taco	170	460	12
Crunchy Taco	170	290	8
Fresco Chicken Soft Taco	150	460	11

Best choices at a Mexican restaurant are to choose your items a la carte. Don't get a mixed meal – pick a taco, and a side dish with mainly rice. Avoid the beans – they are high in potassium. And limit the tomato salsa. Tortillas are good for you, and you could possibly eat a couple extra ones with a dab of butter to fill out your meal instead of another taco or burrito. You probably want to avoid the nachos, just due to the salt and beans they put on them.

TACO BELL® STYLE HARD SHELL TACO
Ingredients:

1.	White Corn Meal	1 Tablespoon
2.	Chili Powder	4 teaspoon
3.	Onion Powder	½ teaspoon
4.	Garlic Powder	1 teaspoon
5.	Paprika	½ teaspoon
6.	Ground Cumin	½ teaspoon
7.	Sugar	½ teaspoon
8.	Dried Minced Onion	1 teaspoon
9.	Lean (90%) Ground Beef	1 pound
10.	Cheddar Cheese, Shredded	¾ cup
11.	Shredded Lettuce	2 cups
12.	Reduced Fat Sour Cream	12 Tablespoons
13.	Hard Taco Shells, Corn	12 each

For the filling, mix together all the spice ingredients except the meat. Stir the spice mixture well to ensure it is well blended. Next, begin browning the ground beef in a large skillet. Once it is completely brown, remove it from the heat. Using a strainer placed on top of a pan (to catch the grease) put the meat in the strainer and soak up the grease with a couple of paper towels (in the pan). Then remove the paper towels and rinse the meat with hot water to remove additional grease.

Return the meat to the pan, and add the spice mixture with 1 cup water. Simmer on low heat for 20 minutes and stir to ensure uniform mixture of spices. Remove from heat before the mixture is completely dry.

Add 2 Tablespoons meat into each taco shell, then top with lettuce, cheese, and sour cream. Serve immediately. 2 Tacos – 1 serving, recipe serves 6.

NUTRITIONAL ANALYSIS PER SERVING:: Calories 376, Protein 23 gm, Carbohydrate 22 gm, Fiber 2.3 gm, Fat 21.7 gm, Saturated Fat 9.6 gm, Phosphorus 320 mg, Potassium 468 mg, Sodium 276

TACO BELL® SOFT TACO LIGHT
Ingredients

1.	White Flour	2 Tablespoons
2.	Chili Powder	4 teaspoon
3.	Onion Powder	½ teaspoon
4.	Garlic Powder	1 teaspoon
5.	Paprika	½ teaspoon
6.	Ground Cumin	½ teaspoon
7.	Sugar	½ teaspoon
8.	Dried Minced Onion	1 teaspoon
9.	Lean (90%) Ground Beef	1 pound
10.	Cheddar Cheese, Shredded	¾ cup
11.	Shredded Lettuce	2 cups
12.	Corn Tortillas (Soft, 6 in)	12 each

For the filling, mix together all the spice ingredients except the meat. Stir the spice mixture well to ensure it is well blended. Next, begin browning the ground beef in a large skillet. Once it is completely brown, remove it from the heat. Using a strainer placed on top of a pan (to catch the grease) put the meat in the strainer and soak up the grease with a couple of paper towels (in the pan). Then remove the paper towels and rinse the meat with hot water to remove additional grease.

Return the meat to the pan, and add the spice mixture with 1 cup water. Simmer on low heat for 20 minutes and stir to ensure uniform mixture of spices. Remove from heat before the mixture is completely dry.

Add 2 Tablespoons meat into each taco shell, then top with lettuce and cheese. Serve immediately. 2 Tacos – 1 serving, Serves 6

NUTRITIONAL ANALYSIS PER SERVING:: Calories 319, Protein 22 gm, Carbohydrate 26.5 gm, Fiber 4 gm, Fat 14 gm, Saturated Fat 6.3 gm, Phosphorus 380 mg, Potassium 435 mg, Sodium 180

(CHINESE) PANDA EXPRESS® AS OF 5/12/13

Product	Calories	Sodium	Protein
Orange Chicken	420	620	15
Mandarin Chicken	250	440	30
Broccoli Beef	120	660	9
Honey Walnut Shrimp	370	470	14
Steamed Rice	490	0	7
Mixed Veggies (Side)	35	260	2
Sweet and Sour Chicken Breast	380	320	15
Cream Cheese Rangoon (3 pcs)	190	180	5
Sweet and Sour Sauce	70	115	0

Best choices at Chinese restaurants are steamed rice, as it is good for a renal diet regardless of your condition. Get a chow mien noodles when you can choose your vegetables – snow peas, string beans, water chestnuts, bean sprouts, and bok choy. Get any sauces on the side. Ask if they have nutrition brochures so you can choose based on sodium and protein content of the food.

ORANGE CHICKEN
Ingredients

1. Water — 1 cup
2. Orange Juice — ¼ cup
3. Lemon Juice — ¼ cup
4. Rice Vinegar — 1/3 cup
5. Orange Zest — 1 teaspoon
6. Soy Sauce, Low Sodium — 1.5 Tablespoons
7. Brown Sugar — 1 cup, packed
8. Fresh Ginger, grated — ½ teaspoon
9. Garlic, Minced — ½ teaspoon

10. Red Pepper Flakes	¼ teaspoon
11. Cornstarch	3 Tablespoons
12. Water	2 Tablespoons
13. Boneless, Skinless Chicken Breast	24 ounces
14. All Purpose Flour	1 cup
15. Black Pepper	¼ teaspoon
16. Olive Oil	3 Tablespoons
17. White Rice, Raw	1 ½ cups

In a saucepan, combine the water, orange juice, lemon juice, rice vinegar and soy sauce, then start to cook over medium heat. Add the orange zest, brown sugar, ginger, garlic, and red pepper flakes to the saucepan and bring the mixture to a boil. Once it is boiling, remove from heat and let it cool for 10-15 minutes.

While sauce is cooling, cut boneless chicken into small (about 1/2 inch) pieces. Place them in a resealable plastic bag and pour 3/4 cup of the cooled sauce into the baggie. Seal the bag and refrigerate for about 2 hours. Once the chicken has marinated for 2 hours, remove from refrigerator. In another plastic bag, mix the flour and pepper. Add the marinated chicken pieces and shake the bag to coat them.

In a large skillet, add the oil and heat on medium. Add the chicken and brown on both sides. Remove the chicken and place on paper towels and cover with foil. Wipe out the skillet and add the reserved sauce. Bring it to a boil again. Mix together the cornstarch and 2 tablespoons water, and add to sauce. Reduce heat to medium low, add back the chicken and cook on low heat for about 5 minutes.

Cook rice according to package directions without additional salt, and serve with chicken. Serves 6, ½ cup rice per person.

NUTRITIONAL ANALYSIS PER SERVING: Calories 582, Protein 29, Carbohydrate 91 gm, Fiber 1.9 gm, Fat 10 gm, Saturated Fat 1.6 gm, Phosphorus 298 mg, Potassium 571 mg, Sodium 284 mg

---

BROCCOLI BEEF

Ingredients

1.	Beef Sirloin, Trimmed, Raw	12 ounces
2.	Broccoli Florets	¾ pound
3.	Canola Oil	2 Tablespoons
4.	Garlic, Minced	2 teaspoons
5.	Cornstarch	1 teaspoon
6.	Water	1 Tablespoon
7.	White Rice, uncooked	1 cup

Beef Marinade Ingredients

1.	Low Sodium Soy Sauce	1 teaspoon
2.	Dry Sherry	1 teaspoon
3.	Cornstarch	½ teaspoon
4.	Black Pepper	¼ teaspoon

Sauce

1.	Low Sodium Soy Sauce	1 1/2 Tablespoons
2.	Honey	1 Tablespoon
3.	Dry Sherry	1 teaspoon
4.	Water	¼ cup

Slice the beef thinly and across the grain. The beef needs to be marinated, so create a marinade with 1 tsp soy sauce, 1 teaspoon dry sherry, 1/2 teaspoon cornstarch and 1/4 teaspoon black pepper. Once you have created the marinade, add the beef slices and stir, then let stand for 10 minutes.

Add the sauce ingredients together in a bowl - 1.5 tablespoons soy sauce, 1 tablespoon honey, 1 teaspoon dry sherry, and 1/4 cup water.

Set the bowl aside, and blanch the broccoli. To blanch, add the broccoli to a small pot of boiling water until crisp - about 2 minutes. Drain and set to the side.

Now, heat a large pan over high heat until a bead of water sizzles when dropped on it. Add the cooking oil and coat the pan. Add the marinated beef and spread it all out over the pan in a single layer. Cook it for about 1 minute, then flip the slices over. Add the garlic to the pan and fry for another 30 seconds. Make sure the beef is no longer pink inside. Pour in the sauce and add the broccoli, then bring to a boil. Pour in the cornstarch (1 tsp) that was dissolved in 1 tablespoon of water, and cook until the sauce boils and begins to thicken.

Cook rice according to package directions without additional salt, and serve with beef. Recipe serves 4, ½ cup rice per serving

NUTRITIONAL ANALYSIS PER SERVING: Calories 453, Protein 24 gm, Carbohydrate 50 gm, Fiber 3.7, Fat 17 gm, Phosphorus 266 mg, Potassium 607 mg, Sodium 322 mg

PANERA BREAD® AS OF 5/7/13

Product	Calories	Sodium	Protein
Egg & Cheese on Ciabatta	390	710	19
Power Breakfast Bowl with Steak	230	310	20
Half Roasted Turkey and Avocado BLT on Sourdough	260	470	16
Half Napa Almond Chicken Salad on Sesame Semolina	340	590	15
Half Tuna Salad on Honey Wheat	250	580	14
Full Classic Café Salad	170	150	2
Full Caesar Salad	310	480	9
Full Honey Tangerine Dressing	100	45	0
Kids Meal – Roast Beef Deli Sand on White	310	730	23
Apple	80	0	0
Plain Bagel	290	460	10
Plain Cream Cheese (1 oz)	100	110	2

Panera bread is great because you can specialize so much of the menu. Many items are high in sodium, but there are great choices. Be wary of the "added" baguette – it contains another 440 mg sodium per piece. Wow. Here is the online calculator:
http://www.paneranutrition.com/?ref=/menu/index.php
Use it before you go to figure out what you can adjust when you order by taking off the added items.

Ask them to not add tomatoes to your meal and you will lower the amount of potassium and phosphorus in your meal.

Product	Calories	Sodium	Protein
6" Oven Roasted Chicken Sub	320	640	23
6" Veggie Delight Sub	230	310	8
Kids Veggie Delight Sub	150	210	6
Kids Black Forest Ham Sub	180	470	10
Kids Roast Beef Sub	200	410	14
Kids Turkey Breast Sub	180	460	10
Oven Roasted Chicken Breast Salad	130	280	19
Roast Beef Salad	140	460	19
B.L.T. Chopped Salad	150	450	10
Tuna Chopped Salad	290	380	14
Honey Mustard Salad Dressing	80	320	1
Sweet Onion Salad Dressing	100	230	0
Egg White & Cheese Melts	150	480	12
Egg & Cheese on 3" Flatbread	190	520	9

At Subway® because you can customize your sandwich so much, you can personalize what type of meal you want. Make sure you don't add pickles and tomatoes. Stick to the kids meal if you can.

NEXT STEPS

1. Go to the websites for the restaurants or fast food places that you like to eat at. Choose the items that are best for you (low sodium, moderate protein) and make yourself a list. Take that list with you when you go there next time.

2. Pay attention to how you feel once you eat a lot of salt versus your normal meal intake. In many ways, you will feel bloated and puffy. Salt keeps a lot of fluid in your body, as well as keeps your kidneys from processing the fluid well.

3. Next time you are out to eat, ask for the sauces on the side and if you can change things about the way the meal is prepared. See that the reaction is positive, especially when you say you have a medical condition that requires some special changes. They don't mind helping.

4. Make a list of quick meals you can take with you on the go – and plan ahead for your next trip so you can take them along.

A few last words before you go out to eat. Planning ahead and asking for changes is the best way to go about getting what you need in a restaurant. Most places will allow you to make changes and to customize your meal. I strongly encourage you to speak up and know what you don't want – tell them no tomatoes, no bananas, etc. You are your own best advocate. And if you feel uncomfortable, make sure they know you have a health condition that requires the changes.

These restaurants that I have included are not the only ones, and they are certainly not the "recommended" places to eat. I want you to be aware of the possible potassium and phosphorus levels so you can make better decisions. You can make your decision about where to eat.

<u>YOU ARE IN CHARGE OF WHAT YOU EAT AND WHERE YOU EAT</u>!

CPSIA information can be obtained
at www.ICGtesting.com
Printed in the USA
LVOW01s2220091016
508058LV00018B/511/P